INCONTINE

OTHER BOOKS IN THE SERIES

1. McKenna You — After Childbirth
2. Laidlaw Epilepsy Explained
3. Meadow Help for Bedwetting
4. Illingworth Your Child's Development in the First Five Years
5. Farquhar The Diabetic Child
6. Illingworth Infections — and Immunisation of Your Child
7. Lewis High Blood Pressure
8. Hampton All About Heart Attacks
9. Tattersall Diabetes — a Practical Guide for Patients on Insulin
10. Farquhar Diabetes in Your Teens
11. Chamberlain Pregnancy Questions Answered
12. Ebner Relaxation and Exercise for Childbirth
13. Porter Understanding Back Pain
14. Moll Arthritis and Rheumatism
15. Milner Asthma in Childhood
16. Clark Adult Asthma
17. Heatley Constipation, Piles and other Bowel Disorders

IN PREPARATION

Chick Drinking Problems
Goldberg Depression
Wood Infertility
Martin Hearing Loss
Thomas Diet and Diabetes
Crisp Anorexia Nervosa
Young Guide to Cancer
Bergman Caring for an Elderly Relative

Patient
Handbook
18

INCONTINENCE

R.C.L. Feneley M.Chir.(Camb.), F.R.C.S.(Eng.)
Consultant Urologist
Southmead Health District
Bristol

J.P. Blannin S.R.N.
Nursing Continence Adviser
Ham Green Hospital
Bristol

Churchill Livingstone
EDINBURGH LONDON MELBOURNE AND NEW YORK 1984

CHURCHILL LIVINGSTONE
Medical Division of Longman Group UK Limited

Distributed in the United States of America by Churchill
Livingstone Inc., 1560 Broadway, New York, N.Y. 10036,
and by associated companies, branches and representatives
throughout the world.

© Longman Group Limited 1984

All rights reserved. No part of this publication may be
reproduced, stored in a retrieval system, or transmitted in
any form or by any means, electronic, mechanical,
photocopying, recording or otherwise, without the prior
permission of the publishers (Churchill Livingstone, Robert
Stevenson House, 1-3 Baxter's Place, Leith Walk, Edinburgh
EH1 3AF).

First published 1984
Reprinted 1986

ISBN 0-443-02855-9

British Library Cataloguing in Publication Data

Feneley, R.C.L.
  Incontinence.—(Patient handbooks; 18)
  1. Urine—Incontinence
  I. Title   II. Blannin J.P.
  III. Series
  616.6'3   RC921.14

Library of Congress Cataloging in Publication Data

Feneley, Roger, 1933—
  Incontinence.
  (Patient handbooks ; 18)
  Bibliography: p.
I. Urine — Incontinence. I. Blannin, J. P. II. Title.
III. Series: Churchill Livingstone patient handbook ; 18.
[DNLM: 1. Urinary incontinence — Popular works. WJ 146
F332i]
RC921.I5F46 1984   616.63   83-27222

Produced by Longman Singapore Publishers Pte Ltd.
Printed in Singapore.

ACKNOWLEDGEMENTS

The authors are grateful to their secretaries, Mrs. M. Butler and Miss M. Bloomfield, who prepared the manuscript, and to Dr. Angela Shepherd, M.D., M.R.C.O.G. for her valuable help and support. They also gratefully acknowledge the help of Mr. Arthur Cottrell, Medical Artist at Southmead Hospital, for the diagrams and figures, and Mr. J.C. Crossley, F.R.C.S., F.R.C.O.G., Consultant Obstetrician and Gynaecologist at Southmead Hospital, for his illustrations.

CONTENTS

1. **Who — me?** 1
   An unmentionable subject 1
   How can the problem be helped? 2
   How many people are affected? 3
   How does urinary incontinence start? 3
   What types of urinary incontinence are there? 4
   How is urinary incontinence cured? 6
2. **The urinary system** 7
   Where does all the urine come from? 7
   The kidneys 8
   The ureters 9
   The lower urinary tract 9
   The communication system 13
3. **How should the bladder work?** 16
   How is the bladder trained? 16
   How often should the bladder be emptied? 18
   How much can the bladder hold? 18
   How fast does the bladder empty? 20
   How is the bladder assessed? 20
   Why does the bladder disturb some people at night? 22
4. **What makes the bladder misbehave?** 24
   How much should I drink? 25
   Does it matter what I drink? 26
   Can drugs affect the bladder? 27
   Does anxiety affect the behaviour of the bladder? 28
   Does the menstrual cycle affect the bladder? 29
   How does the menopause affect bladder function? 29
   How does sexual activity affect the bladder? 30

	Does bowel function also affect the bladder?	31
	Can baths affect the bladder?	32
	Does the climate influence bladder function?	32
	Does putting on weight cause bladder problems?	33
5.	**What can I do?**	34
	What part of the system has failed?	34
	How is the fault traced and how can this be corrected?	35
	A problem of panic	36
	The problem of life in retirement	38
	An irritable bladder	39
	A case of bedwetting	41
	The problem of stress incontinence	42
	The frustration of the 'after-dribble'	45
	The urinary incontinence which cannot be controlled	46
6.	**Uncontrolled urinary incontinence**	48
	When do I need to wear protective pants and pads?	48
	How will the nurse decide which aids are best for me?	49
	What aids are available for men?	53
	How do I take care of my appliance?	
	How do I protect my skin?	57
	Urinals (bottles)	58
	Are there any other aids?	59
	What is a catheter?	60
Further reading suggestions		66

1. WHO — ME?

Urinary incontinence is for many people an embarrasing subject, and a book about it is hardly the type of reading matter you will often see in a prominent place in most homes. Yet there must be so many households where the problem of those uncontrollable leaks of urine occurring at inconvenient moments and in inappropriate places is a cause for some concern.

Perhaps everyone, if they are absolutely honest, is aware of such mishaps at some time in their life, but few would ever admit that they were frankly incontinent. They might accept that they had a little accident, which suggests that the leakage was just one of those unfortunate events that should never have happened. For some people, these little accidents can become an ever-increasing burden. So often those who suffer in this way try to ignore their problem, rather than take any positive steps to correct the situation. In fact, the problem is only recognised when, in utter despair, they realise that they can no longer hide the truth from others.

An unmentionable subject

Urinary incontinence is not a problem that should be suffered in silence. Ignorance is not bliss for those who have to endure this miserable state. The sudden, unexpected loss of self-control is a humiliating experience that arouses a deep sense of helplessness and shame. Many people feel far too embarrassed to mention their problem, even to their own doctor, because it takes courage to admit to being wet. Haunting fears and unncessary worries arise about the future. All too often the problem is concealed by one means or another and even the everyday pleasures of life may need to be severely modified.

How can the problem be helped?

The first task is to remove the attitude of mystery and taboo that surrounds the whole subject of urinary disorders and to replace them with a better understanding of the human waterworks. For most people, the ability to control the passage of urine is such a natural event that little attention is given to the matter. Even the healthy act of passing urine is often described in vague terms that no foreigner could ever understand. 'Micturition' somehow sounds such an indecent word to describe the simple task of emptying the bladder, that it has to be couched in terms such as 'spending pennies' or 'going for a leak'. The exercise is a very personal matter and a routine is developed for it. This routine tends to become a habit and some habits can he harmful and difficult to change. A surprising number of people are fully aware that they have always had a weak bladder and they have to visit the toilet more often than their friends. They are quite prepared to put up with that, so long as they retain full control. Unfortunately for some, their bladders start to control them, dominating their thoughts and causing anguish and loss of self-confidence. Anxiety merely makes the situation yet more intolerable. Questions arise which they are afraid to ask. Many people could be helped if they had more idea of how their urinary system worked. Most equipment is supplied with a useful instruction manual, which gives simple hints on what to do when something goes wrong. Perhaps the midwife forgot to leave one with the new arrival!

How many people are affected?

Urinary incontinence is a very common disorder and many more men and women are troubled than one would expect. There are probably over two million people in the United Kingdom who suffer from the problem to a greater or lesser extent and many of them are leading busy active lives. It is surprising how many complain that they have had to give up playing games, such as tennis or taking exercise by jogging or dancing. Surveys on over 5000 young healthy women showed that about 50% of them were aware of occasional episodes of incontinence, but they did not seek advice, either because of their embarrassment or because they did not consider the problem to be abnormal.

Incontinence imposes a particularly heavy burden on elderly people. In those over 65 years of age, about one in every ten women and a slightly smaller proportion of men suffer from occasional urinary leakage. Few of them seek or receive any expert advice about their problem and yet they may take considerable trouble to hide their distress. Any excursion from the home has to be carefully planned, so that they can make sure that they can easily reach a toilet. Some unfortunately become too afraid to leave the security of their home.

The Year of the Disabled in 1981 focused attention on the needs of those who are handicapped and who require the care and help of others. There are over three million of them living in private homes in Britain and many suffer conditions which render them incontinent. Public awareness may have been aroused and at least the need for providing special facilities, such as amenable toilets, was recognised. But the question may well be asked whether sufficient attention has yet been taken to ease the many practical problems that their urinary incontinence presents to them or their families.

How does urinary incontinence start?

The familiar story is one of a sudden, unanticipated dribble of urine and this is followed by another and another, at shorter and shorter intervals. A little detective work is required to discover just what is happening. Did the leakage occur before or after visiting the toilet, or was it just 'out of the blue'? Was it associated with sudden exertion or did it arise during sleep at night? Careful enquiry is necessary to identify the pattern of the urinary loss and certain types are well-recognised.

What types of urinary incontinence are there?

The most common type of urinary incontinence, affecting men and women of all ages, is the one associated with a desperate feeling, as if the bladder is about to burst. In fact, the bladder will not burst whatever one may think, but surely most people will appreciate that feeling when they need to make a 'run for it'. They shuffle their feet, cross their legs, waiting for an opportunity to make a discreet exit, holding on like mad. Unfortunately, they are not exactly sure what they are holding on to and sometimes they just have to let go. Some find that their legs will not carry them fast enough and

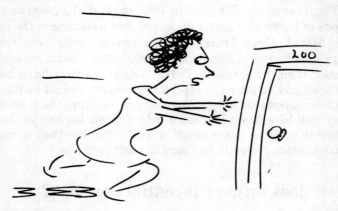

Urge incontinence

the inevitable leak of urine occurs. This is a demoralising problem and it is termed appropriately 'urge incontinence'. So often, those who experience the disorder react instinctively by restricting the amount of fluid that they drink, particularly when they pluck up courage to venture on a social outing, and they make quite sure that they visit a toilet whenever the opportunity arises. In fact, such a regime can only make matters worse and it does nothing, either to restore normal bladder function or their shattered morale.

Another common type of incontinence is the urinary leakage that occurs on coughing, laughing or sneezing. This is essentially a problem that affects women and one lady admitted that she laughed so much that 'tears ran down her legs'. This type is termed 'stress incontinence', because it is associated with physical straining or sudden exertion. The urinary leakage starts with a few drops of urine that stain the underclothes and so often the instinctive reaction is to wear

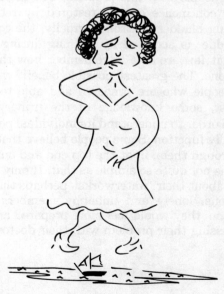

Stress incontinence

some form of protection or to carry a spare pair of pants. Again, this response to the problem does nothing to strengthen the bladder control and it is, therefore, not surprising that the final results are so depressing.

Both 'urge' and 'stress' incontinence illustrate common types of urinary leakage, which tend to get slowly worse if urgent steps are not taken to improve bladder control. Far too many people struggle on stoically with minor little leaks for years, until their morale is finally broken by a major catastrophe. At that point, they seek urgent advice for an instantaneous cure, only to be bitterly disappointed to discover that no such magic exists.

How is urinary incontinence cured?

There are a variety of different methods of curing incontinence, because there are so many different causes. For the majority of people with this problem, who are otherwise fit and active, continence can be restored by retraining and strengthening bladder control. Normally, the control of the urinary bladder is acquired by training during early childhood, so that few are able to remember how they achieved that milestone. The greatest possible benefit will be gained by those people who are prepared and able to help themselves. First, some knowledge of the urinary system is essential, in order to understand its individual parts and how they normally function. Some people believe that water runs straight through them, in at the top end and out at the bottom, but it is not quite so simple as that. If only more people knew more about their 'waterworks', perhaps there would be fewer anxious, lonely and unhappy members of society. Hopefully too, they would feel more prepared and confident about discussing their problem with their doctor.

2. THE URINARY SYSTEM

Where does all the urine come from?

Urine is formed by the kidneys and normally this process continues throughout life. The urinary equipment is conveniently divided into two parts, namely the upper urinary tract with the kidneys and ureters and the lower urinary tract, by the bladder and urethra (see Fig. 1).

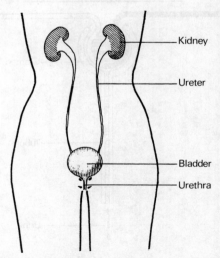

Fig. 1 The urinary system

The kidneys

There are two kidneys, one in each loin, but the body can survive efficiently for a full lifespan on only one. The kidneys act as an intricate filtration system for the blood. A large volume of blood is streamed through the kidneys every minute by the heart, which acts as the pumping station. The main vessels, or arteries, conduct the blood to the kidneys and these divide into smaller and smaller branches as they enter the kidney, to deliver the blood to about 2 million minute filters called glomeruli. In these glomeruli, there is a delicate membrane, rather like a filter paper, which separates the blood on one side from the kidney tubes or tubules on the other (Fig. 2). Water and the dissolved chemicals in the blood pass across this membrane into the kidney tubules, whilst the blood cells and proteins are held back. After filtering the blood in this way, the kidney tubules select out and exchange the essential ingredients, which the body requires, from the excess water and

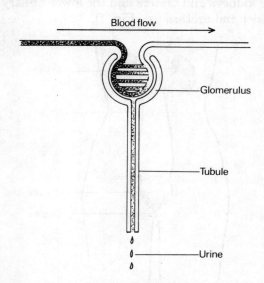

Fig. 2 Diagram to illustrate filtering of blood by glomeruli

waste products, which can be discarded in the urine. A healthy person, on a well-balanced diet, forms between two and three pints of urine (1200 — 1800 ml) in a 24-hour period.

The ureters

Urine formed in this way passes through the collecting system in the kidney to reach the ureters, which act like supple drainpipes propelling their contents towards the bladder. At the lower end of each ureter, where they enter the bladder, there is a delicate mechanism which acts like a valve. This ensures that the urine passes in only one direction from the kidney into the bladder and it prevents urine passing back from the bladder towards the kidney. This mechanism provides an important protection for the kidneys. For example, it prevents an infection in the bladder from washing back up the ureters and hence spreading the infection to the kidneys.

The lower urinary tract

The bladder

The bladder collects the urine from the upper urinary tract, stores it and then empties the contents through the urethra, to discharge it from the body. The bladder has a remarkable ability to change its size, rather like the balloons which are blown up at children's parties. Its walls consist of muscle and elastic tissue, so that it can distend to store urine and contract to empty it. Bladders appear to come in a variety of sizes, some small and some large. A small bladder has to be emptied more frequently and the owners of this type often complain of having a weak bladder. On the other hand, the large bladder does not need to be emptied nearly so often. How envious some people are of the hearty character with a 'camel-like bladder', seemingly of infinite capacity, who can drink five pints of beer without having to move from his perch by the bar! Many people are rather surprised and perhaps a little shocked if asked how much they can hold in their bladder. In fact, bladder capacity is an important measurement, although perhaps few would consider it to be one of the 'vital statistics' of the body.

The urethra

Urine escapes from the bladder by passing along the urethra. In women the urethra is a short passage, just over 1 inch in length, whereas in men it is much longer, as it reaches to the end of the penis (Fig. 3). The male urethra also conducts the seminal fluid, which is discharged from the region of the prostate gland. This gland surrounds the urethra just below the bladder and as the prostate enlarges with age, it can occasionally interfere with the flow of urine.

Although there are marked differences in the length and shape, the actual mechanisms that control the opening and the closing of the urethra are very similar in both men and women. An incontinent person often refers to the need for a 'new washer' in the system, to prevent their urinary

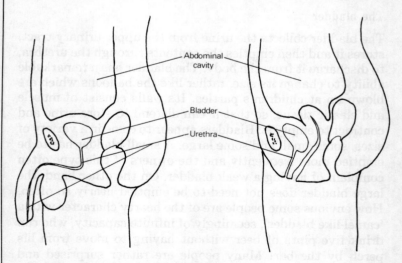

Fig. 3 The male and female lower urinary tract

leakage. There are in fact two 'washers', or to give them their correct description, sphincters, which normally close the urethra. One sphincter is situated where the urethra leaves the bladder and this is referred to as 'the bladder neck sphincter'. The second one is about 1 inch below this and it is called 'the external sphincter'. Both sphincters are very important in controlling the passage of urine, but the external sphincter is the only one which can be consciously controlled and, therefore, in this book it will be called 'the voluntary sphincter'. The voluntary sphincter acts rather like a noose around the urethra and can be tightened to grip the passage or loosened to open it (Fig. 4).

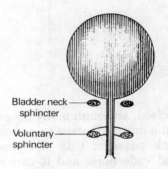

Fig. 4 The sphincters which close the urethra

On either side of the voluntary sphincter, there is a large mass of muscle termed 'the pelvic floor muscle'. This forms a type of broad hammock, slung across the cavity of the pelvis from the front to the back, and it supports the whole contents of the abdominal cavity. The urethra passes through the front part of this muscle, whilst the bowel or rectum passes through the back part before it reaches the anus (Fig. 5). In women, the vagina or birth canal is situated between these two structures and, during childbirth, the baby's large head can stretch and weaken the pelvic floor muscle. This muscle, like the voluntary sphincter, can be

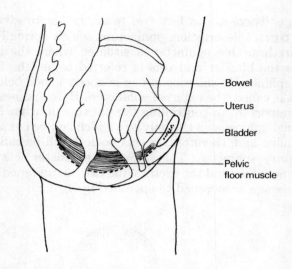

Fig. 5 The pelvic floor muscle

consciously exercised, although many people are not aware of this. In fact, the muscle is used to prevent wind passing through the back passage; this can produce rather an embarrassing and rude noise and it can be prevented by pulling-up and contracting the muscle. The pelvic floor muscle exerts a type of pinching action on the urethral passage. By working with the voluntary urethral sphincter, it should be possible to contract or pull-up on these muscles and stop the flow of urine when the bladder is being emptied. In this way, the passage of urine can be interrupted and started again.

The urethral opening on the surface of the body is called the external urethral meatus. This is tucked away in women, just in front of the vaginal opening, and it can be difficult to find. In men, the opening is at the tip of the penis on the part known as the glans.

The communication system

In order to recognise when the bladder is full or when it is empty, there has to be a very efficient communication system between the lower urinary tract and the brain. This is a very complicated part of the equipment and it consists of many nerves, which are rather like telephone wires that carry messages to and fro between the bladder and the brain. The bladder, the urethra and the structures around

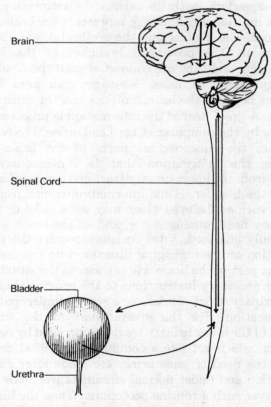

Fig. 6 The communication system

the urethra, such as the pelvic floor muscle, are wired up with a very large number of fine nerves, which are connected to the spinal cord. Some of the nerves carry information in the form of electrical impulses from these structures to the spinal cord and others carry information back in the opposite direction. In the spinal cord there is a relay station, through which all the information passes to and from the brain (Fig. 6).

The whole system may be compared to the communications system in a large commercial organization. The headquarters, with its various departments on every floor of a multi-storey building, represents the brain and the spinal cord. The bladder and the urethral mechanisms are, so to speak, the provincial branches of the business organization; and they are connected with the head offices by many telephone lines. Messages can pass in both directions between the branch offices and the central headquarters. A great deal of the information is processed automatically by the computer at the head office. The computer represents the subconscious parts of the brain and it processes the information that is continuously being received from the lower urinary tract and sends information back to the bladder. Some information comes from other sources, such as the eyes which may see a toilet or the ears which may hear running water, and all the reports have to be carefully analysed. Vital decisions require the personal deliberation of the managing director, who represents the conscious part of the brain. He can assess the situation and send any necessary instructions to the provincial offices.

The urinary tract works on a very similar pattern of communication. For the greater part of the time, the function of the lower urinary tract is controlled by centres in the brain, which act like a computer. The vital decisions, such as the need to pass urine, are made after conscious deliberation and under normal circumstances little time is wasted over such a routine procedure. When the bladder is full, the message is received by the brain and emptying proceeds at an appropriate time and place. Any interference or damage to this communication system at any level, whether it is at its periphery, in the computer or in the conscious part of the brain, may grossly disturb the co-ordination of the lower urinary tract, which depends on an intact nervous system.

3. HOW SHOULD THE BLADDER WORK?

The behaviour of the bladder varies so widely from one individual compared to another that it is difficult to say what is 'normal'. What one person may consider to be normal can be quite abnormal for another and, in any case, most people recognise that their own bladder can be quite unpredictable at times. Furthermore, these matters are just not discussed because the subject is usually considered to be rather a disagreeable one. It can, therefore, be difficult for someone to find out what is considered to be normal and a few basic facts may help to clarify the picture and to answer some of the questions which people are anxious to know. Perhaps it is best to start at the beginning and consider how the bladder is first trained.

How is the bladder trained?

All babies are incontinent. The bladder fills and empties automatically, but by the age of three years most children have gained control during the day and, by the age of five, the majority will also be dry during the night. The child has to learn how to recognise the sensation of bladder fullness and to associate this with the need to pass urine when 'sitting on the potty'. Mothers may assist this learning process by turning on a tap, so that the child associates the sound of running water with passing urine. The mother may be fastidious about her training method, 'potting' the child regularly every two to three hours during the day, or she may adopt a far more easy-going approach, allowing the child to learn by trial and error. At first, children often have very little warning about the need to empty the bladder and they commonly experience a sense of urgency to do so without delay. At one moment they are playing happily with their toys and at the next they are running to reach the toilet in time. Little accidents are not uncommon at this stage. Their control soon improves, as they learn to postpone emptying the bladder until a convenient opportunity arises, but some learn this faster than others. Bladder control is termed 'a conditioned reflex', because it is acquired by training. This conditioning of the bladder is controlled by the development of the nerve connections between the brain and the bladder, which are incomplete at birth, and it does need to be properly maintained throughout life.

The child also has to learn to empty the bladder completely. If one watches young children pass urine, some have to strain quite hard to start the emptying process, but this should not be necessary when they have developed full control. Emptying of the bladder should proceed until the last drops of urine have been drained from the system, but some children are far too impatient to wait that long.

During this stage of bladder training, problems can develop in children. They may not store urine well enough or they may not empty their bladder completely. These things are usually very transient, but sometimes they can continue into later life. As every schoolteacher knows, some children have difficulty in learning how to postpone the need to empty the bladder and they suffer from a frequent and urgent sensation of wanting to do so, even at the most inconvenient times. This problem may persist into adult life and the usual complaint is one of having a weak bladder. The ability to store urine and then to empty it at a convenient time does vary a great deal and it can depend on the way that the bladder has been trained to behave. Anyone could train their bladder to empty every half-hour, but such a habit would be extremely inconvenient. Many factors do influence the habit, apart from mere convenience. The disgrace and fear of being wet are natural instincts that were probably developed during the training period in childhood.

How often should the bladder be emptied?

The majority of people pass urine between four and eight times a day and they establish a regular pattern that is convenient for them. The frequency of passing urine depends on two factors, namely how much can the bladder hold and how much urine is produced during the day and night.

How much can the bladder hold?

The bladder has two essential functions; to store urine and then to empty its contents at a convenient time and place. Urine enters the bladder continuously in a steady trickle throughout the day and night from the upper urinary tract and its only means of escape is through the urethra. The bladder acts as a storage tank for the urine, so long as the urethra remains closed. The rate of filling does vary, but an average rate is about 2 fluid ounces (60 ml) per hour. A normal healthy bladder should be able to hold between one-half and a full pint of urine (20 fl.oz.) at its best. Thus a period of at least five hours should be possible before the bladder needs to be emptied. The bladder usually holds its largest quantity during a night's sleep. If a person sleeps for eight hours and produces 2 fl.oz. of urine per hour, the bladder will need to hold 16 fl.oz. (480 ml), if sleep is to remain undisturbed. During the daytime, the actual amount of urine that is held in the bladder before emptying is necessary does show a wide variation.

How is the bladder emptied?

The sensation of fullness is the usual signal that leads to voiding of urine or, in other words, emptying of the bladder. This sensation is not always particularly reliable. There are times when the bladder feels full, yet it contains far less than its actual capacity. The sight of the toilet or the sound of running water may stimulate an awareness of the bladder and raise a false alarm. Most people will recognise occasions when they feel that they would like to empty the bladder, but something happens to distract them, such as a telephone call or a doorbell ringing, and quite a long time may pass before they feel the need to pass urine again. This illustrates how the bladder can be suppressed by unexpected circumstances and, in the meanwhile, more and more urine is being stored.

To empty the bladder the urethra must open. As explained in the previous chapter, the urethra is fitted with a voluntary sphincter, supported on either side by the larger mass of pelvic muscles, and both these mechanisms can be consciously controlled. The sphincter and the pelvic muscles grip and pinch the urethra respectively, to keep it closed during the period of bladder storage. To open the urethra, these muscles must relax, thus releasing their grip on the urethral passage and this triggers the bladder to contract. The situation is rather like blowing-up a toy balloon and holding the spout between the thumb and forefinger. When the grip is released, air rapidly escapes and the balloon collapses. There are times when delay or hesitancy may be experienced in starting the flow of urine, because this sphincter is slow to relax. Only a small amount of urine has to leave the bladder before the sensation of fullness disappears, but the computer mechanism in the brain should ensure that voiding continues until all the urine has been discharged. The urinary stream can be interrupted voluntarily, if the sphincter and pelvic muscles are tightened up during the emptying process and then, by relaxing them again, the stream is re-established.

How fast does the bladder empty?

Young boys enjoy a spirit of competition and some will even compare how far they can 'shoot' their stream of urine up a wall or over a five-bar gate! The rate of flow of the urine does vary a great deal and it tends to become slower with age. Many people notice that their urinary stream varies from time-to-time and some become very self-conscious about the matter. The flow of urine tends to be slower when the bladder is emptied during the night or in the early morning, compared to other times during the day. Some people find it very difficult to pass urine in a public toilet, particularly when there is a long queue or when they are very apprehensive about something.

The rate of flow of the urinary stream can now be measured by means of modern electronic meters. Women tend to have much higher flow rates than men and can empty a full pint of urine from their bladders in less than a minute. Young men pass their urine faster than the older ones. The rate of urine flow does depend on the amount of urine that is passed. If the bladder is only holding a small quantity of urine, the stream tends to be little more than a dribble, whereas if the bladder holds a good half-pint or more, the flow is much faster. As one gentleman explained, his flow was much better after three pints of best bitter. A good average flow rate in a woman is about 15 ml (½ fl.oz.) per second, which is equivalent to 300 ml (10 fl.oz.) in 20 seconds. A good average rate for a man is around 10 ml per second, or 300 ml (10 fl.oz.) in 30 seconds. The rate of flow, however, is much lower than this if the amount of urine passed is less than 150 ml (5 fl.oz.).

How is the bladder assessed?

A simple practical way of assessing the behaviour of the bladder involves keeping a chart, which records the frequency and the volume of urine that is passed. The only requirements are a wrist watch or a clock to record the time and a suitable jug that measures the quantity of urine passed on each occasion, in either fluid ounces or millilitres. A pint jug holds 20 fl.oz. or about 600 ml (Fig. 7). Every time that urine is passed, a note is kept of the time and the amount of urine voided during a 24-hour period. An example of a normal record is shown in Fig. 8 and this illustrates a number of features. The individual had to pass urine 5-6 times during the day. A large amount of urine was passed first thing in the morning at 7.00 a.m. after a night's sleep and then, during the day, the amounts varied widely, between 120 ml (4 fl.oz.) and 360 ml (12 fl.oz.). If the record is kept for a few days, a pattern for that person emerges. There are certain times, such as arriving at work, during the lunch or tea-break and before going to bed at night, when it

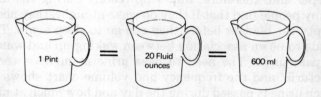

Fig. 7 Capacity of a pint jug

Day	Day-time time/volume (ml or fl.oz.)						Night-time
1	7 am	9 am	12.30 pm	4 pm	9.15 pm	11.30 pm	
	450 mls	120 mls	250 mls	350 mls	300 mls	150 mls	
2	7.30 am	12.30 pm	2.30 pm	6.15 pm	11.15 pm		
	400 mls	320 mls	140 mls	250 mls	360 mls		
3	7.15 am	12 m.d.	2 pm	5 pm	7.45 pm	11 pm	
	420 mls	350 mls	120 mls	250 mls	200 mls	180 mls	

Fig. 8 A normal record of urine passed in one day

is that person's custom to empty the bladder. The chart also shows the total amount of urine that is passed during the day and, on average, a normal person will produce about 1500 ml (50 fl.oz.), or about 1 ml per minute.

Why does the bladder disturb some people at night?

Most people are able to sleep through the night without disturbance from the bladder, but it is not uncommon for some, particularly the elderly, to find that they have to pass urine at least once — and occasionally twice or more — during the night. The chart does help to analyse this habit. Sleep may be disturbed because the bladder is full of urine and needs to be emptied. On the other hand, a person may be a very light sleeper and, therefore, wakes up readily during the night. Many people find that if they do wake at night, they need to empty the bladder before they can go to sleep again. There tends to be an association between waking up and wanting to pass urine. The need to pass urine at night is termed 'nocturia' and the frequency and volume chart shows how much urine is passed during the day and how much at night. Some elderly people produce more urine at night than they do by day. The chart in Figure 9 shows this very clearly. During the day this elderly man only passed 600 ml, but during the night he passed 900 ml and it is, therefore, not surprising that sleep was disturbed. Many elderly people

Day	Day-time time/volume (ml or fl.oz.)					Night-time			
	8.30 am	12	4 pm	7.15	10 pm	1 am	3.15	4.30	7 am
1	140	100	120	140	100 mls	250	300	200	150

Fig. 9 Frequency and volume chart

find that they do not sleep as heavily as they did when they were younger. Sleep in fact seems to become a series of 'cat-naps' for about three or four hours at a time. They probably do not need as much sleep as they did when busy at work and they should not be too worried if that occurs.

4. WHAT MAKES THE BLADDER MISBEHAVE?

Everyone can surely recall certain occasions in their life, when the behaviour of their bladder has caused some inconvenience. Maybe the frequency of passing urine was increased or there was a sense of extreme urgency about finding a toilet, which caught them unawares. A night's sleep may have been disturbed by the need to empty the bladder, particularly after a memorable party with a plentiful supply of drinks. Usually such experiences are rapidly forgotten and well before a visit to the doctor is considered necessary. On the other hand, the appearance of blood or the onset of pain when passing urine do suggest that something is more seriously wrong and the doctor should be consulted without delay.

Alterations in the familiar routine of passing urine may be due to a number of factors. Probably we all know a friend or a relative who always seems to be making visits to the toilet. If a person is worried about the number of times they are 'going', the frequency and volume chart described in the previous chapter does help to analyse what is happening. Many people discover for the first time how their bladder is behaving. Frequency of bladder emptying is not only related to the bladder size, but there are a number of everyday factors which can affect its function.

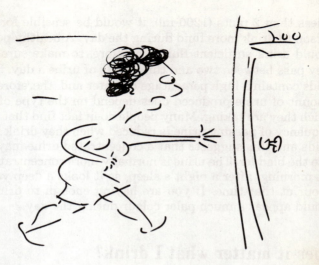

Urgency

How much should I drink?

This is a very common question and there is no doubt that eating and drinking habits do vary a great deal. Some people make a regular habit of drinking a glass of water when they clean their teeth in the morning and they always have another glass at lunch and at dinner in the evening, whilst others merely rely on cups of tea or coffee during the day. The body requires food to supply it with energy and, like any source of energy, waste products are produced. Many of these waste products are discharged from the body in the urine. If they are dissolved in about a pint of water, they produce a very concentrated urine, which appears a deep yellow colour and smells rather strong. A much healthier output of urine is between two and three pints, (1200-1800 ml) a day. The chart is a very useful way of checking how much urine a person produces in 24 hours. If it is less than 2 pints (1200 ml), it would be sensible for that person to drink more fluid during the day. A healthy person should drink sufficient fluids therefore, to make sure that they pass between two and three pints of urine a day. Some foods contain a high percentage of water and, therefore, the amount of urine produced does depend on the type of diet which they are taking. Many people do in fact find that their frequency of passing urine is reduced when they drink more fluids and this suggests that a concentrated urine may irritate the bladder. The urine is normally more concentrated in the morning, after a night's sleep, so it looks a deep yellow colour at that time. If you are having enough to drink, it should appear a much paler colour during the day.

Does it matter what I drink?

Certain beverages, such as tea and coffee, do have a mild diuretic action, which means that they increase the output of urine by their effect on the kidney. This increased output of urine may cause a more frequent need to empty the bladder and some people are more sensitive to their action that others. Alcoholic drinks can have a similar effect on some people. Men commonly admit that if they drink a pint of beer, they need to pass a quart of urine. They become self-conscious and embarrassed by the number of visits that they have to make to the 'gents'. Some women too discover that certain alcoholic drinks appear to irritate the bladder and they take care to avoid them.

The prudent individual wisely experiments with various drinks, to investigate their effect on the bladder. Perhaps by avoiding the cup of tea or coffee before going to bed, there will be no need to get up in the middle of the night to pass urine, or by avoiding that second cup of tea or coffee during the day and taking a glass of fruit juice instead, the frequency of micturition may be reduced. Barley water is the traditional drink, which people with a bladder disturbance are advised to take, and it is well worthwhile trying this as an experiment. A useful recipe for barley water is as follows:

1 teacup pearl barley
4 pints boiling water
2 lemons, 6 oranges
Demerera sugar to taste

Put barley in a large saucepan, add boiling water, simmer over a low heat with the lid on for one hour. Strain water from the barley, adding the rind of one lemon and three oranges. Allow to stand until cold. Strain off the rinds and add the orange and lemon juice. Keep in a refrigerator.

If the frequency of passing urine becomes an inconvenience, it is much wiser to drink more rather than less fluid.

Can drugs affect the bladder?

A number of drugs nowadays are used deliberately to make people pass more urine. Some of these are extremely powerful and rapidly produce an increased output of urine. They are used for a variety of reasons, mainly to remove the excess fluid from the body. People often refer to them as their 'water pills'. They do stimulate the need to pass urine more often and it is advisable to take them in the morning, otherwise sleep can be disturbed at night.

Other drugs in common use may have some side effect on bladder function. For instance, drugs used in the treatment of asthma or chronic bronchitis, or those prescribed for high blood pressure can alter the normal function of the bladder. It would be wise to discuss this matter with the doctor, if a change in the bladder behaviour does become apparent when you are taking any drugs.

Does anxiety affect the behaviour of the bladder?

Anxiety or any emotional upset can affect a person's normal pattern of bladder behaviour. Most of us are conscious of the need to pass urine before an important event, such as an interview for a job or even a visit to the doctor. This, of course, is one of the many problems with regard to the bladder itself. When people start to worry about their bladder, their frequency so often increases and the problem is compounded in a vicious circle. Bereavement is certainly one of the most distressing experiences of life and elderly people can suffer a considerable disturbance of bladder function at such times. Sympathetic help from friends and relatives can provide them with the greatest comfort. A sudden shock of any type may have a similar effect on the bladder.

Retirement from work involves a radical change in life-style for most people and the necessary readjustment may cause an alteration of bladder behaviour. During a busy programme of work, there may be little time for paying attention to the bladder, but the retired life can alter that. The extra cups of tea or coffee during the day and the convenience of the toilet in the home, may start to set a pattern which can be difficult to break. The visits to the toilet set a trend of 'a little and often' and the more often the bladder is emptied, the more often the need arises.

Gradually the storage capacity of the bladder is reduced, the urine flow dwindles and the sleep is disturbed at night. Some may call it 'the old man's disease' and blame the prostate, so that a visit to the doctor becomes necessary. For a small proportion of men, the enlargement of the prostate may be the cause, but how often the problem may have been preventable by disciplined control of the bladder perhaps we shall never know. The prostate is essentially a sexual gland, but by that stage of life sexual activity has so often diminished or been neglected for years.

Does the menstrual cycle affect the bladder?

The hormonal changes that occur during the menstrual cycle may influence the function of the urinary tract. The vagina and the uterus (or womb) are situated just behind the urethra and bladder, so that it is not surprising that variations in bladder function may arise during the cycle. The inner lining of the urethra is particularly sensitive and occasional urinary leakage is noted by some women during the week before a period. Some women find that their bodies retain fluid at this time and they may notice slight swelling of the ankles, tightness in the breasts and a feeling of lower abdominal distension. At the same time they may find that they pass less urine than usual. During a period, the use of tampons may cause irritation to the urethra in some women, but they usually recognise this for themselves.

The increasing size and weight of the uterus during pregnancy can press on the bladder and cause an increase in the frequency of micturition, particularly during the early months. The birth of the baby stretches and may weaken the pelvic floor muscles and cause some loss of bladder control in the form of stress incontinence. This will be described in more detail in a later chapter, but normally the problem rapidly settles, particularly if attention is paid to post-natal exercises.

How does the menopause affect bladder function?

Following the menopause, there is a sharp reduction in the level of female hormones in the body and this causes changes to occur in the skin and the lining in and around both the vagina and the urethra and they lose their natural elasticity. Irritation of the urethra and the loss of the elastic tissue in the bladder may cause increasing frequency of passing urine. The use of hormone tablets or a hormone cream applied to the vagina can be beneficial in this condition and the doctor may prescribe this.

How does sexual activity affect the bladder?

Some women experience an increased frequency of passing urine following sexual intercourse. This may be due to the fact that the urethra and bladder lie very close to the vaginal wall, and the external urethral and vaginal openings are immediately adjacent to each other. As a result, intercourse may directly irritate the delicate urethra, particularly if there is a lack of adequate vaginal lubrication. Unfortunately, bladder symptoms can make women understandably apprehensive about intercourse and this only makes matters worse. Apprehension reduces the vaginal lubrication and causes the pelvic muscles to contract, so that a vicious circle develops.

Cystitis is a common complaint, which may be associated with sexual activity. Cystitis is a misleading description, because it suggests that there may be a urinary infection. In fact, many women who suffer from cystitis following intercourse do not have any evidence of infection. The problem can play havoc with any attempts to establish a normal sex life and many women complain that it has ruined their marriage. The condition used to be termed 'honeymoon cystitis', implying that the problem arises following the onset of sexual activity, but that is not necessarily the case. Cystitis sometimes arises following a change of sexual partner, which suggests that it may in some cases be related to the male seminal fluid. Seminal fluid contains various substances, which can be absorbed through the vaginal wall and certain constituents are known to influence bladder function. Women who suffer from this complaint are often advised to make a habit of passing urine immediately after intercourse, but this can hardly promote the pleasure and relaxation that they should enjoy.

Cystitis following sexual intercourse is probably related to a number of factors and a certain amount of detective work on the part of the individual is not without benefit. Lack of vaginal lubrication may be one factor that has to be considered. The position used for intercourse is another and adjustment of this may remove the irritation to the urethral orifice or to the urethra itself. A pillow placed under the buttocks provides an answer for some women. If the seminal fluid is thought to be a possible cause of irritation, temporary use of a contraceptive sheath may be tried. If bladder symptoms do occur, a plentiful supply of drinks, a hot bath and a hot-water bottle may prove helpful. Antibiotics are occasionally necessary, but so often they are followed by a thrush infection of the vagina, which is a miserable complication. The simple answers are always the best.

Does bowel function also affect the bladder?

Bowel and bladder function are indeed closely linked. Messages from the bowel and the bladder travel in the same nerve bundles back to the brain. Sometimes the messages seem to become short-circuited and there can be difficulty in distinguishing between a full bladder and a full bowel. Frequency of micturition in some elderly people can be alleviated by making sure that they empty the bowel properly. The bowel does tend to become lazy at times and constipation is a common cause of bladder symptoms. Careful attention should be paid to maintaining a regular bowel action, but this does not have to be every day. Most people find that they develop their own regularity and this varies from one or more times a day to once every second or third day. Your diet is important and you will benefit by having enough roughage in the form of bran and wholemeal bread, but an adequate fluid intake is always essential. If you do not drink enough, bowel motions becomes hard and difficult to pass.

Can baths affect the bladder?

Regular baths are important for normal hygiene, but you should be careful not to add substances which may cause irritation to the skin around the genitalia. Strong antiseptics can cause irritation to the sensitive skin in this area, but it is surprising how often they are regularly used by some people. Even bubble baths or heavily chlorinated water in a swimming pool can cause cystitis in some women.

The normal secretions under the foreskin in men can be a source of chronic irritation to a sensitive part of the penis. These should be removed by retraction of the foreskin when taking a bath or a shower. If the foreskin becomes difficult, the doctor should be consulted.

Does the climate influence bladder function?

Temperature and humidity influence the amount of water that is lost from the body via the kidneys. In a dry, hot climate more water leaves your body through the lungs in your breath and from the skin in the form of sweat. Under these conditions, your urine output can be greatly reduced and you need to pass urine infrequently. Some people who suffer from a weak bladder find that they have no problems when they are enjoying the sun around the Mediterranean. On returning to a temperate climate, particularly in a cold, wet atmosphere, the water loss is readjusted, so that more is lost through the kidneys. This often explains why people returning from the tropics to the United Kingdom experience quite a marked increase in the frequency of passing urine.

Does putting on weight cause bladder problems?

An increase in weight in middle age is due to the laying down of fat in various parts of the body. A great deal of fatty tissue is formed inside the abdomen and this increases the weight of the contents, causing pressure on the bladder and the pelvic floor. The additional weight resting on the bladder may decrease its capacity and cause a more frequent need to pass urine. The pelvic floor muscle has to support the contents inside the abdomen and any increased weight on this can weaken the controlling mechanisms around the urethra. Stress incontinence can become a problem in women who have put on too much weight.

5. WHAT CAN I DO?

The onset of urinary incontinence is a horrifying experience and for those who are leading an active life it introduces a major threat. Ominous fears rapidly develop about the future and the emotional response clouds any rational approach to the problem. A logical plan is essential, in order to analyse what is happening. In the earlier chapters I attempted to describe the various structures in the urinary tract and how they normally function to control the storage and passage of urine. The human waterworks is a complex piece of equipment and many factors can influence its delicate balance. When any piece of intricate machinery fails to perform normally, it is an advantage to have a definite plan to identify the fault. Three basic questions need to be answered:
1. What part of the system has failed?
2. How can this be traced?
3. What can be done to correct the problem?

What part of the system has failed?

There are three components in the urinary tract, which have to be considered when the system develops a leak. The bladder is the storage tank, which holds the urine and then empties at convenient times and in appropriate places. The urethral passage is the escape route for the urine from the bladder and the structures in and around this apply the mechanics to open and close the pipeline. Thirdly, the nervous system provides the computer and all the necessary wires to co-ordinate the function of the bladder and the urethra and it also allows the system to be consciously controlled by the brain. Urinary incontinence may be due to malfunction of one or more of these basic components. Under normal circumstances, each part depends on the function of the other two parts, so that the whole system works in unison. When urinary leakage occurs, a methodical check must be undertaken. Is the leakage due to a failure of the bladder to store an adequate amount of urine? Are the urethral mechanisms working properly to close the passage during urinary storage or to open adequately during bladder emptying? Is the nervous system working properly to give sufficient warning that the bladder is full and to allow bladder emptying to be postponed until a convenient time?

How is the fault traced and how can this be corrected?

The bladder holds a variable amount of urine, but if for some reason its storage capacity is reduced, urine has to be passed more frequently and very often there is a sense of urgency about doing so. This can lead to the problem of 'urge incontinence', which is perhaps the most common type of incontinence to affect men and women of all ages. Urge incontinence is the urinary leakage that occurs with an extremely urgent feeling of wanting to pass urine. Every normal person knows that they can reach a point at which their bladder can hold no more and, when this arises, increasing urgency is experienced to empty the bladder as soon as possible. Most people have been taken by surprise at some time in their life, when they have had to hurry home to reach the toilet in time. Under extreme conditions, a small dribble of urine may leak from the bladder before the toilet is reached and, as soon as that happens, the sense of extreme urgency may pass away for a short while.

For those people who suffer from urge incontinence, these occasions recur with increasing regularity. They may complain that they have always had a 'weak bladder' and this usually means that they have a small bladder capacity. If that is the case, they can check the amount that the bladder holds by keeping a chart, as described in Chapter 3. Most people who experience frequency, urgency and urge incontinence tend to pass small volumes of 180 ml (6 fl.oz.) or less on each occasion and, for some reason, they have lost the ability to hold larger volumes. This may be variable, so at times they pass a large volume and at other times a small one. This suggests that the bladder capacity is perfectly normal, but there are times when they just cannot inhibit the urge to pass urine. On the other hand, some people always have a small bladder capacity, which never reaches a normal volume, and this loss of bladder capacity may require further investigation.

The frequency and volume chart does help to assess the problem in more detail and a few examples may illustrate this. When incontinence is the major cause of the complaint, any episodes of urinary leakage are noted on the chart with a 'W'.

A problem of panic

Mrs J. (aged 54) was becoming very concerned about her bladder problem. The frequency of passing urine during the day was interfering with her life, to the extent that she was becoming afraid to take part in any social activity, in case she was suddenly 'caught short'. Her greatest fear was that she was going to be incontinent, so she had taken to using a sanitary pad, just to avoid any possible disaster. She kept a chart very carefully and measured all the volumes in millilitres (this is shown in Fig. 10).

Day	Day-time time/volume (ml or fl.oz.)											Night-time
	8 am	8.45	9.30	10.15	11.15	12 md	1.30	4.0	7 pm	9.15	10.30	6 am
1	150 mls	30	30	40	50	30	60	80	120	100	50	300 mls
	7.30	8.15	9.00	9.45	11 am	12.15	1.15	4.15	6.45	10.15		5.30 am
2	80	60	50	30	40	50	40	100	100	150		400 mls

Fig. 10 Mrs J.

On analysing her record, the most important feature was that the bladder could hold over ½ pint of urine at certain times. In her case, this occurred during the early hours of the morning, after about seven hours sleep. On one occasion she actually passed 400 ml and, therefore, the bladder capacity could be perfectly normal. Her greatest problem was during the morning, when she was passing urine in small volumes nearly every hour. During the afternoon, she had a part-time job, which kept her very busy, and the frequency was less troublesome. On adding up the total amount of urine that she passed throughout a 24-hour period, the actual volume was less than two pints. In fact, she admitted that she was afraid to drink too much, in case this made her problem worse. A noticeable point was the complete absence of any recorded incontinence of urine and, when asked about this, she admitted that she felt that she was going to lose control, although in fact at no time did she do so while she was keeping the chart.

Mrs J. was very surprised when it was brought to her attention that she had a normal bladder capacity and she quite agreed that she was not drinking very much because she thought that would only make matters worse. Furthermore, she could sleep for about seven hours without disturbance, but when she did wake up, she usually had to get up to pass urine.

Mrs J. naturally asked what could be done about her problem. She was told that she had a normal bladder size and, therefore, it was very unlikely that she had any serious problem so far as that was concerned. She was advised to drink more fluids and to attempt to hold the bladder for longer periods before going to the toilet. In fact, she had always considered that it was wise to pass urine whenever an opportunity was available. She started retraining her bladder by the clock method. At first, she visited the toilet every two hours during the day, then she gradually lengthened this until she could hold urine for three-to-four hours. When she felt as if she wanted to empty the bladder, she was advised to set the kitchen timer for three minutes and she then tried to postpone her visit to the toilet until the bell rang. Some people find that an egg-timer can be used in a similar way and they practise holding on until all the sand has run through. After a little practice, Mrs J. was beginning to regain her confidence and after six months, she announced that she had full bladder control again. On one of her visits, Mrs J. mentioned that her problem had started soon after her mother died. Her mother had suffered a mild stroke and she had become incontinent following that. Mrs J. had looked after her mother until she died and her worst fear was that she was going to become incontinent like her.

The problem of life in retirement

Mr H. was aged 68 and he was becoming anxious about the frequency with which he had to pass urine. On occasions he was becoming aware of extreme urgency to empty the bladder and a small dribble of urine occurred before he managed to reach the toilet at times. This stained his underpants and he was concerned that the problem was going to become worse. He passed urine with a pretty good flow and he noticed that he was in and out of the toilet faster than most of his contemporaries. He kept a chart and this is shown in Figure 11. When questioned about the chart, he pointed out that he usually experienced a slight dribble of urine when there was only a small amount of urine to pass.

Day	Day-time time/volume (ml or fl.oz.)							Night-time
	7.30 am	9 am	10 am	2 pm	3.30 pm	7 pm	11.15	3 am
1	400 mls	W80 mls	W60 mls	300 mls	W100 mls	250 mls	300 mls	350 mls

Fig. 11 Mr H.

He found that the sound of running water from the kitchen taps was enough to set him 'running', as he put it. At other times, he only had to think about his bladder and he could not delay micturition. The total amount of urine that he was producing amounted to about 3 pints (1800 ml) per day. Since he had retired, he had been drinking more tea and coffee at home and he always had a cup of tea before going to bed. He usually had to get up once at night to empty his bladder. He had to admit that he was not taking very much exercise.

Mr H. was advised to adjust his habit of drinking so much tea and coffee. He avoided drinking a second cup and instead had a glass of fruit juice. He also stopped drinking tea before going to bed. Mr H. started taking some more exercise during the day and he found that he managed to sleep some nights without having to get up to pass urine. On occasions, he could wake up in the morning and pass 500 ml of urine with a good flow, and thus he certainly had no cause to worry about his bladder capacity.

An irritable bladder

Mrs T. (aged 64) complained that she was always going to the toilet and her sleep was disturbed every night. This was a great trial for her, as she found that she felt so tired during the day. Her problem had started after she had had an abdominal operation and she had never been able to regain her bladder control following that. Her chart is shown in Figure 12.

Day	Day-time time/volume (fl.oz.)								Night-time			
	7 am	9	11	12.30	2	4.30	6	8.30	10	12.30	3 am	5 am
1	3	3	4	2	2	3	2	4	2	3	2	4

Fig. 12 Mrs T.

The essential feature of Mrs T's chart is that her bladder never held more than 4 fl.oz. (120 ml) at any one time. It was quite clear that her bladder capacity was reduced for some reason or other and she was advised to have some further investigations. She had a very irritable bladder and the storage capacity was considerably reduced at all times.

An irritable bladder can be due to a number of different causes and medical advice is required to discover the reason for this condition. The bladder may be extremely sensitive, so that it sends too many messages to the brain, warning the person that it is full when in fact it is not. An infection in the urine is one common cause of this. The bladder does not distend and thus fails to act as an adequate storage tank. Sometimes, as the bladder begins to fill, the muscle in its wall starts to contract before the person is ready to empty the bladder. If a contraction does arise, the bladder pressure rises quite rapidly and in this way it forces urine down the urethra. Urine can only flow from the bladder through the urethra to produce a leak, if the bladder pressure is greater than the pressure closing the urethra. This condition has been termed 'the unstable bladder'. Modern methods of studying the pressure changes in the bladder and the urethra have provided a considerable amount of information regarding bladder disorders. Mrs T. was referred to the hospital for her investigations, which included special studies of her bladder behaviour and an examination of the bladder, known as a cystoscopy. Following these, she responded to treatment with some tablets and she only wished she had not ignored her problem for so long.

A case of bedwetting

Mr S. (aged 72) was very distressed. He discovered that he had wet the bed one night and he felt quite shocked about this. He had been noticing for some while that his frequency of passing urine had increased and he was having to strain to micturate. His urinary stream was little more than a dribble and he had to wait for some while before he managed to start the flow. His chart is shown in Figure 13.

Day	Day-time time/volume (ml)										Night-time		
	7.45	9.15	11 am	12.30	1.45	2.30	3.45	5 pm	7 pm	9.15	12 mn	3.15	5 am
1	100	80	100	100	80	60	80	100	126	100	120	120	W110

Fig. 13 Mr S.

The main point about Mr S. chart is that he is passing 'a little and often'. In fact, he never managed to pass more than 120 ml (4 fl.oz.) at any one time. His bladder capacity seemed to be reduced and he gave a very good account of the very poor urinary stream that he experienced. Mr S. required further investigations. These showed that he was not emptying his bladder properly. The urethral passage was not opening adequately and he was retaining a considerable amount of urine in the bladder. His type of urinary leakage is termed 'overflow incontinence'. In retrospect, Mr S. should have consulted his doctor earlier. He had noticed the increased frequency and he had been straining to pass urine for some while. He had an operation to open the neck of the bladder and he was delighted to find that he could pass his urine again as well as he had in his younger days.

No book on urinary incontinence can be complete without mention of the problem of bedwetting. This is a subject that is normally a problem in childhood, but there are a few adults who continue to wet the bed regularly at night. Some experience frequency, urgency and urge incontinence by day and bedwetting at night and they very often have a small bladder capacity. During a period of eight hours sleep, between 12 and 15 fl.oz. (360-450 ml) of urine may be produced. If the bladder normally only holds less than 10 fl.oz. (300 ml), it is not surprising that the bladder needs to be emptied at night. Some young adults find that they only wet the bed after they have been drinking a large amount of fluid. They can sometimes help themselves a great deal, by trying to increase the bladder capacity during the day. If they can learn to 'hold on' and postpone passing urine for long and longer periods, they can train their bladder to store a larger quantity. In fact, the subject of bedwetting has been extremely well covered by another book in this series, by Dr Roy Meadows entitled *Help for Bedwetting*.

The problem of stress incontinence

Mrs K. (aged 47) had, as she described, almost reached the end of her tether. She had been aware for some while that she had the occasional leakage of urine and this occurred whenever she coughed, laughed or sneezed. She smoked about 20 cigarettes a day and she tended to have a 'smoker's cough', which was becoming more troublesome. She recently had a severe cold and the combination of sneezing and coughing had made her urinary leakage very much worse. In fact, she had spent an evening with a friend and, to her horror, when she stood up from the chair, she noticed that there was a small damp patch on her skirt and the seat of the chair. In fact, she had been wearing a

Day	Day-time time/volume (ml)									Night-time
	8.15	9 am	10.30	11 am	12	2.30	6 pm	7 pm	10 pm	11.30
1	300	W	50	250	W30	300	200	W50	250	100

Fig. 14 Mrs K.

sanitary pad for protection, but this was saturated. She kept a chart of her frequency and the episodes of incontinence and this is shown in Figure 14.

The chart shows that Mrs K. had a very normal bladder capacity. She could hold large volumes of urine in the bladder before she had to visit the toilet. Her urinary leakage only occurred on exertion. She was asked whether she could stop and start the urinary stream when emptying the bladder, but she had never tried to do this. When she did attempt to do the exercise, she found that it was almost impossible. Perhaps the urinary stream slightly slowed up, but it did not stop. She could pull in the back passage to stop wind from passing and she was advised to try pulling up a little harder and to practise this exercise. By pulling up on the back passage, she was learning to raise the pelvic floor muscles, which were described as a type of hammock in Chapter 2. If she pulled up very hard, she could feel it lifting up this hammock and pulling in the front of the tummy, below the belly-button. She was told to pull up and let go and then encouraged to repeat this about twenty times. Once she had learnt this exercise, she started practising it in regular sessions throughout the day. Whenever she passed urine, she tried to start and stop the stream and gradually she found that she was beginning to stop the flow of urine. She could start it again by relaxing the muscle.

Apart from her pelvic floor exercises, Mrs K. had to take herself in hand in other ways. Her cough was undoubtedly becoming a problem and her smoking habit was clearly injurious. She was advised to give up smoking and fortunately she was one of these strong-minded individuals who decided to do that immediately. When she did cough, she was told to pull up the pelvic floor muscles at the same time and, in that way, to close the urethral passage. She admitted that she had been putting on weight over the past few years and this, of course, weakened her pelvic muscles. She had given birth to three children when she was younger and her last baby was a big one and, on reflection, she admitted that her problem had started shortly after the birth of that child.

By hard work and sheer determination, Mrs K. learned to use her pelvic floor muscles properly, cured her chronic cough and reduced her weight. Over a period of three months, after really conscientious effort, Mrs K. discovered that she could avoid her problem of stress incontinence.

Stress incontinence in women is a common type of urinary leakage. It occurs on exertion, when your tummy muscles are pushing hard. This causes pressure which is immediately transmitted to the bladder and forces out a small volume of urine down the urethra. Normally on straining, the pelvic floor muscle should automatically tighten to prevent this leakage from occurring. As explained in Chapter 2, the voluntary sphincter and the pelvic floor muscles grip and pinch the urethral passage and, in this way, keep it closed during bladder storage. If the pelvic floor muscle has been weakened, it fails to tighten sufficiently to prevent urine escaping from the bladder. Childbirth may damage these muscles, but normally recovery should take place so long as post-natal exercises are regularly practised. Women who have had four or more babies are more liable to suffer from this form of incontinence. The weakness may not be revealed immediately, but the pelvic muscles can tend to grow weaker with age, particularly if the person puts on weight as they approach the menopause. The best way to check if these muscles are working properly is to stop the urinary stream whilst emptying the bladder. Most men can perform this exercise without any difficulty, but there are a large number of women who have little or no idea that they possess such a muscle.

In some cases of stress incontinence, the pelvic floor muscles and the ligaments that support the uterus, or womb, are so severley damaged that remedial exercises alone are not sufficient to cure the problem. If this is the case, the doctor will probably advise a specialist opinion. In a proportion of women, an operation may be necessary.

Nevertheless, a very large proportion of women can be cured by conscientious remedial exercises.

The frustration of the 'after-dribble'

Mr L. (aged 52) was very distressed because he noticed that he was beginning to wet his clothes. He discovered that after passing urine he would walk away from the toilet, only to find that there was a tell-tale patch of urine, about the size of a 50p piece, on his trousers. This stained his underclothes and the trousers, which was both upsetting and most embarrassing. He kept a chart of his frequency and the amount of urine that he passed and this showed that there was no problem regarding the amount that he could hold in the bladder. He had begun to think that he was developing a problem with his prostate, as his father had experienced this type of trouble.

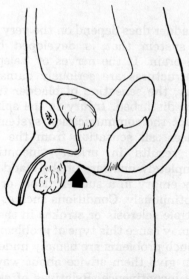

Fig. 15 Gentle pressure over the base of the urethra to empty the remaining drops of urine

An 'after-dribble' of urine is a common complaint amongst all age groups and it is due to the fact that the urethral passage is not emptied completely before leaving the toilet. This type of leakage is not a sign of any serious abnormality, but it means that the muscles around the urethra are not emptying the tube properly. For some reason, which is not fully understood, the muscles become lazy and do not squeeze out the last few drops from the pipeline. Although this is a frustrating problem, it usually improves without special treatment and it is not a disorder that progressively deteriorates. The best way to prevent the problem is by applying gentle pressure with the fingers over the base of the urethra, to compress it and to push out any remaining drops that may be present (Fig. 15).

The urinary incontinence which cannot be controlled

Control of the bladder does depend on the very complicated communication system that is developed between the bladder and the brain. If the nerves or 'telephone wires' between these structures are seriously damaged for one reason or another, the sensation of bladder fullness or of emptying may be disturbed. Injury to the spinal cord can completely disrupt the communication system and, under these circumtances, all sensation from the bladder disappears, which results in urinary incontinence. The individual is completely unaware of the bladder emptying. The bladder may empty in a sudden flood, or it may just dribble away continuously. Conditions such as spina bifida in children, multiple sclerosis or strokes in the elderly, are examples which may cause this type of problem. People who are affected by such problems are usually under the care of doctors, who can give them advice about ways of coping with the urinary incontinence. Relatives of elderly people are only too aware of the problems of urinary incontinence and there are many ways in which they can be helped. Urinary leakage must be controlled to avoid damage to the skin and there is a wide range of aids and appliances, which can be considered. It is important to seek professional advice on these matters and some of the available methods are described in the next chapter.

6. UNCONTROLLED URINARY INCONTINENCE

Urinary incontinence that cannot be controlled does require careful investigation by the doctor. Particular attention is needed to ensure that the kidney function is not placed at risk of damage. Apart from the medical aspects, the individual desperately wants good practical advice, so that a suitable and acceptable method of coping with the urinary leakage is provided. This chapter outlines the various ways that can be considered and illustrates the advice which the nurse or continence adviser, with special experience of the problems, is able to give.

When do I need to wear protective pants and pads?

Protective pants and pads are aids for the incontinent patient to use. They are not a cure for the problem, though far too often a pair of pants are regarded as such and may even lead some people to accept their incontinence. A better understanding of the various causes of incontinence is essential. The continence adviser will want to know if pelvic floor exercises have been practised regularly every day or if an honest attempt has been made to retrain the bladder. Regaining continence is not easy; it requires extra effort.

There needs to be strong motivation and, in time, confidence will be regained by the ability to overcome the problem.

Is the pad being worn 'just in case'? A trial period without pads and pants is a useful exercise, but a time should be chosen when the individual can relax and be comfortable at home. It is easy to rely upon the pad, which gives a feeling of security and lessens the need for personal effort. Some people are quite surprised how much control they do have and this is a great step in building up confidence.

There are some people, who have been assessed by the doctor and do have an intractable incontinence. They do need to wear pads and a pad should be chosen, which is capable of absorbing the urinary leakage, so that embarrassing episodes are avoided.

As the design of pads and pants improves, so too does the complexity of selection. Each type is developed with a particular need in mind. The right pants in the wrong situation can spell disaster. It is well worthwhile seeking the advice of the nurse at the health centre.

How will the nurse decide which aids are best for me?

For those with urgency and urge incontinence, the first priority must be that the pants can be quickly removed. If the amount of urinary loss is small, a small absorbant pad is all that is required.

The young woman with stress incontinence does need to continue to feel attractive and should not be made to feel different, so the nurse should offer a modern style in a pretty fabric. The urinary loss, once again, is usually small so a small pad is perfectly adequate. The not-so-young with stress incontinence also needs similar consideration. Many elderly ladies would prefer a bloomer style, but unfortunately it can be difficult to secure a pad with this type.

For the male patient who needs to wear pads, the nurse

should offer Y front pants, which will hold a pad securely; trunk style underpants are not suitable for this purpose because they are too loose.

The handicapped patient, with total incontinence, will need a pad able to absorb large amounts of urine. There are pads that are able to absorb such quantities, but they cannot absorb urine at the rate at which it is passed. To obtain greater absorbancy, the pad can be cupped in the hand prior to putting it in position (see Fig. 16).

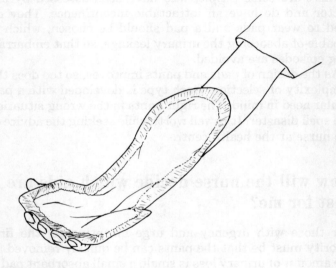

Fig. 16 Cupped pad

A common mistake is to put several layers of pads together without removing the plastic insert sheets and, of course, this does not increase absorbancy. It should not be assumed that a large pad is necessarily more absorbant. Small, less bulky pads are being developed now which will have much higher absorbancy.

There are many considerations in assessing the suitability of the pants for the individual's requirement:

Marsupial pants (see Fig. 17)

The marsupial pant with a waterproof pouch to hold a pad in position is a very popular design. Urine can pass through the material and is absorbed by the pad, but the material next to the skin remains dry, provided the pad is not worn too long and becomes completely saturated. Many people find this hard to accept, feeling that once urine has contaminated the pants, they are no longer clean. To overcome this, they put the pad next to the skin and in this way they destroy the effectiveness of the design.

These pants come in all sizes and the hip and thigh must be measured to ensure a snug fit. However, they are not recommended in cases of:

1. *Poor dexterity.* Two hands are needed to insert the pad.
2. *Mental alertness.* Good co-ordination is required.
3. *Vaginal/urethral discharge.* Odour may be a problem with this design.
4. *Faecal incontinence.*
5. *Poor hygiene.* The person must be capable of washing the garment.
6. *Poor motivation.* There is no incentive to change the pad.

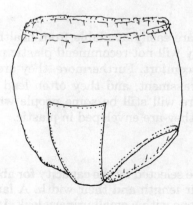

Fig. 17 Marsupial pants (with pouch)

Lightweight stretch pants (Fig. 18)

These lightweight stretch pants give adequate support to keep the pad in position. These have fewer contra-indications and are acceptable to both men and women. They also have the added advantage that the choice of plastic backed pads is not limited to the one recommended by the manufacturer. The cost is low, washing is easy and they dry very quickly. The elderly, who don't take easily to flimsy pants, may wear their own style over the top. It is not a good idea to wear several pairs of ordinary pants at once, because this will only lead to increased odour and overheating, which can lead to soreness and skin rashes.

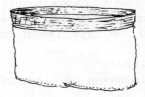

Fig. 18 Lightweight stretch pants

Plastic pants

Plastic pants are easily available from health centres. The nurse generally will not recommend plastic pants, because they cause discomfort. Furthermore, they are noisy, which causes embarrassment, and they often lead to skin problems. But there will still be some people who do not feel secure unless they are enveloped in plastic.

Pads

Pads need to be selected by the capacity for absorbing urine, as well as their length and their width. A large pad is unnecessary to cope with a small urinary leak. It is not a good policy to wear a single pad, allowing it to become soaked over many hours. It is better to use a small pad and change frequently. Urine only smells when it becomes stale and is exposed to the air, allowing bacteria to grow. The bulkier pads are generally more useful at night.

The disposal of pads is a problem for many people. It is wise to find out about the policy in your district regarding the disposal of soiled pads. Some authorities provide special bags for this purpose. Soiled disposable items should be wrapped in newspaper before disposal. Few pads are truly soluble, so avoid flushing them down the toilet.

Supply

Pads and pants are available from your local health centre or clinic. These are unlikely to be issued without first consulting the doctor. The community nurse will not normally deliver them to the home, unless she has to make a call for treatment.

Incontinence aids can be purchased from specialist shops, which sell aids for the disabled, and some larger chemists. Some manufacturers do offer a postal service.

What aids are available for men?

An appliance is a very satisfactory method of management for most men, but some may not be anatomically suited to a device. Gross obesity, a retracted penis or a scrotal hernia may make the device less satisfactory or even impossible to fit. Such an appliance is usually made up of several components (Fig. 19).

There is a waist belt with groin straps and a sheath with a bag to collect the urine.

Great care must be taken in the fitting of the appliance; if it is too tight it may cause swelling of the penis; if it is too large it may be uncomfortable and lead to leakage of urine and the collecting bag may fill with air. It is not advisable to acquire an appliance through newspaper advertisements,

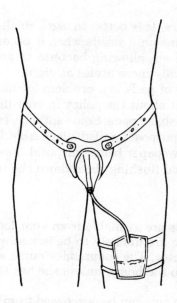

Fig. 19 Pubic pressure urinal in place

because they seldom suit the individual need. The doctor's advice should be sought and he will usually make an appointment, so that a careful fitting can be made. A prescription can then be obtained for further supplies from the local chemist.

Pubic pressure urinals

This is the most complex type of appliance, because of the number of component parts (see Fig. 20). It has various sizes of flanges and sheath diameters and different cones for those who can and cannot walk. It is made of latex rubber and has either plastic disposable bags or latex washable bags. Although the pubic pressure urinal is suitable for all types of uncontrolled incontinence, it may not be suitable for people with poor eyesight, limited manual dexterity or for those who are mentally confused.

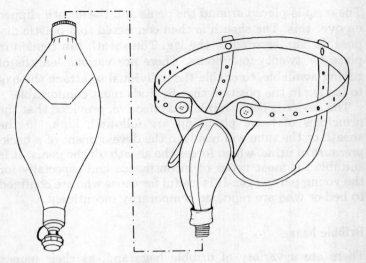

Fig. 20 Pubic pressure urinal

The condom urinal

This is a very satisfactory aid, consisting of a sheath which is attached to a collecting bag (Fig. 21). The design has considerably improved in recent years; the most satisfactory of these is secured by an adhesive strip. The skin should be shaved to ensure that the adhesive sticks firmly.

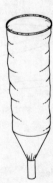

Fig. 21 Sheath (condom)

The strip is placed around the penis and the sheath slipped on over this. The sheath is then connected to a plastic disposable bag, secured to the leg. The sheath can remain in place for twenty-four hours. There are various lengths of tubing available, to enable the individual to attach the bag to his leg in the position that he finds most comfortable.

The device is both simple and effective, provided that the principles of basic plumbing are followed; kinks in the sheath or the tube will result in the development of a backpressure of urine, which forces the sheath off the penis. It is suitable for most types of incontinence and especially for the young paraplegic. It is useful for those who are confined to bed or who are rendered temporarily incontinent.

Dribble bags

There are a variety of dribble bags and, as their names suggests, they are designed for those who have a minor dribbling incontinence (Fig. 22).

The appliance may consist of a plastic bag on a waist band, which is disposable. Others have a washable belt with

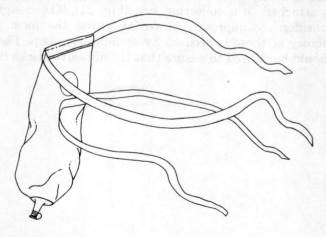

Fig. 22 Dribble bag with tapes

a lined waterproof pouch to collect the urine. Disposable absorbant pouches are also available, which are secured in position over the penis by wearing pants which provide adequate support.

How do I take care of my appliance? How do I protect my skin?

The appliance must be washed daily in the following manner:
1. Take the appliance apart.
2. Rub the flange and cone with salt to remove any film that may be present.
3. Wash well in warm soapy water.
4. Rinse and dry well.

It is necessary to have three appliances, which can be used in rotation and cared for in the manner described above. They should last about a year.

Skin care

When a person is first supplied with an appliance, it is advisable to become gradually accustomed to its use, wearing it for two hours only on the first occasion. When the appliance is removed, the skin should be inspected for soreness on the penis, groins and hips, taking particular care to observe the underside of the penis, as a pressure sore may develop. A practice should be made of observing the condition of the skin each time the appliance is removed. If soreness is observed, the appliance should not be worn until the skin has completely healed. Soreness may become a problem, but the doctor can supply a non-greasy barrier cream, which will alleviate this. The genitalia should be washed daily and dried thoroughly but gently. Do not use too much talcum powder.

Urinals (bottles)

Most people are familiar with the traditional glass urinal. This type of bottle is now available in lightweight polythene. These bottles have a flattened base, which makes them suitable to be used in bed. People often worry about spillage of urine when using a bottle, but this can be avoided by using a non-return valve, which fits into the neck of the bottle (Figs. 23a and 23b). The chairbound patient often finds it difficult to use the conventional type of bottle, because spillage so easily occurs due to the angle at which the bottle has to be held. A useful alternative is a plastic disposable bottle with a rigid neck, which is easy to handle and, when fitted with a non-return valve, the risk of accidents is considerably reduced (see Fig. 24).

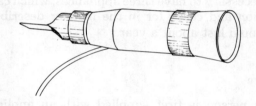

Fig. 23a A non-return valve

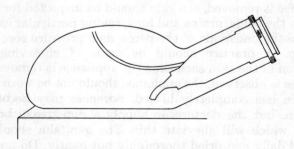

Fig. 23b Urinal with non-return valve in position

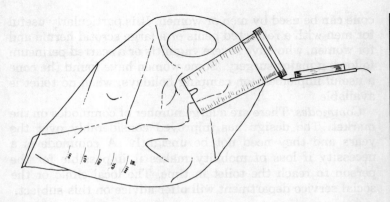

Fig. 24 Disposable plastic bottle

There is also a disposable bag with a built-in valve, which is ideal for use whilst travelling; these bags are completely watertight and discreet. A box of ten is even smaller than a box of tissues.

Are there any other aids?

Besides the appliances which have been described, there are various urinary collection receptacles, especially manufactured for women who are unable to reach a toilet.

St. Peter's boat is an egg-shaped dish with a handle, which may be slipped easily between the legs.

Slipper bed-pan is shaped like a slipper and the pan has a flat bottom and a hollow handle, through which it can be emptied.

Feminal urinal is a collapsible urinal, which can be tucked into a handbag. It consists of a plastic frame, shaped to fit the female anatomy, and a disposable plastic bag is attached for the urinary collection. With practice, the urinal can be used when standing, sitting or lying.

The cone is a special piece of equipment, designed for those who have difficulty in directing the flow of urine. The cone can be used by men or women. It is particularly useful for men with a retracted penis or a large scrotal hernia and for women, who have severe vaginitis or a scarred perineum following major surgery. Some women have found the cone a useful implement on camping holidays, when no toilet is available.

Commodes. There are a large number of commodes on the market. The design has improved considerably over the years and they need not be unsightly. A commode is a necessity if loss of mobility makes it impossible for the person to reach the toilet in time. The local clinic or the social service department will offer advice on this subject.

What is a catheter?

A catheter is a hollow tube, which is passed through the urethra into the bladder. At the tip of the catheter is a balloon, which can be filled with water and thus retains the catheter in position (Fig. 25).

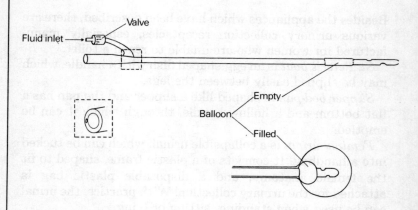

Fig. 25 A self-retaining catheter with a balloon at its tip which can be filled with fluid

When is a catheter used for urinary incontinence?

The doctor decides to use a catheter when the other methods of managing urinary incontinence are considered unsuitable. People who require to be nursed in bed for some reason and who are unable to use urinals can be kept dry and free from skin sores by means of a catheter. This form of urinary drainage can be extremely useful for those who have no control over their bladder and, indeed, for those who have to look after them. Continuous dribbling incontinence is a most depressing condition, both for the individual concerned and for those who care for them, and the catheter can provide a convenient answer to the problem. The care of an elderly person who has become bedridden can become greatly eased for relatives by this means.

How shall I look after the catheter?

Good catheter management does depend on the individual or the family understanding the principles which are involved. Most people appreciate the basic plumbing principles. Water only drains downhill and, if a blockage develops in the pipe, the water will cease to flow. Thus,

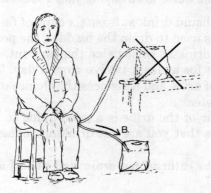

Fig. 26 'A' shows the incorrect and 'B' the correct position for the drainage bag

every effort should be made to ensure that the tubing is free from kinks and the collecting bag is placed well below the level of the bladder (Fig. 26).

A daily bath is advisable when a catheter is used. This keeps the genitalia and the catheter clean and prevents sores from developing. If it is not possible to have a daily bath, the outside of the catheter around the urethral opening should be washed carefully with soap and water twice a day. When a bath is taken, the catheter can be detached from the collecting bag and a small spigot, or bung, can be inserted into the end of the catheter.

Can a catheter cause urinary infection?

The presence of a catheter in the bladder does tend to give rise to a urinary infection. Such infection will normally remain in the bladder and is not associated with any serious risk. An infected urine does appear cloudy, but it is unlikely to make the person feel ill. It is important that the catheter is changed regularly by the doctor or nurse, so they are able to keep a check on this matter.

Why does the nurse keep saying that I must drink more?

Everyone should drink at least six cups of fluid each day. If a catheter is used to drain the bladder, the person is usually advised to drink at least twice this amount, so it is a good plan to aim for at least twelve cups a day. This ensures a good flow of urine and it reduces the chance of any blockage in the catheter.

The colour of the urine is a good guide to observe. Dark urine means that you are not drinking enough.

Why does the catheter not drain well when I am constipated?

The lower part of the bowel is close to the bladder and, when loaded with a solid stool, it tends to obstruct the catheter and prevent proper drainage. A well-balanced diet is very important when the bladder is drained by a catheter. If you ask at the clinic they will advise you about what you should eat.

Is it possible to have intercourse when a catheter is used?

Intercourse is possible for women, but certainly not ideal. It is virtually impossible for men and it may cause serious damage to the urethral opening at the end of the penis. If the problems are experienced with regard to sexual function, it is wise to discuss this with a doctor or nurse. An alternative method of catheterisation may be more appropriate. Some people are now taught to catheterise themselves and, under certain circumstances, this has proved very successful. Another alternative is a supra-pubic catheter. This is placed directly into the bladder, through the skin of the lower abdomen, and the doctor may suggest this.

I have a catheter. How can I keep this a secret?

All too often, it is only too obvious that a person has a catheter because the urine drains into a collecting bag, which cannot be hidden. This is really not necessary. There are a variety of collecting bags, of varying capacity, which can be worn under the clothes. One type may be worn suspended on a belt around the waist or fitted into a pocket in a special pair of pants. Some collecting bags can be attached to the thigh or the calf and, in this way, hidden from view. These methods do provide a discreet way of hiding the collecting bag, so that it is no longer obvious to others. For women who like to wear trousers, it is more convenient to have the collecting bag attached to the lower leg, which makes it easy to empty the bag without undressing (Fig. 27).

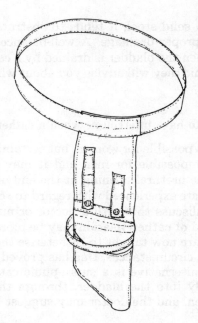

Fig. 27 Holster belt

Can I use the bag more than once?

The majority of bags are made of plastic and are disposable, but the bag may be used more than once at home, as long as it is washed thoroughly in soapy water and allowed to dry. It is not advisable to leave the bag soaking in antiseptic solution overnight. Such solutions can be effective over a short period, but if left overnight it may encourage the growth of bacteria rather than preventing it. A supply of bags may be obtained on prescription.

I understand that some people can be taught to catheterise themselves. When may this be suggested?

Self-catheterisation is offered to those people who have difficulty with emptying the bladder. This may be caused by a bladder that does not contract or a urethra that fails to relax and open to allow the urine to escape.

The technique of self-catheterisation is simple. The nurse usually starts by explaining some basic anatomy and the site of the urethral opening. The opening of the urethra in women is difficult to see and the catheter may need to be positioned by using a mirror. A catheter may be passed quite simply whilst sitting on the toilet. If careful hygiene is observed, there should be no fear of introducing infection. The hands should be carefully washed before and after catheterisation. The catheter is cleaned by washing in soapy water, rinsed and dried thoroughly. It is then stored in a clean container, but the use of antiseptics should be avoided.

FURTHER READING SUGGESTIONS

Incontinence and its management. Edited by Dorothy Mandelstam, 1980. (Croom Helm, London).

Incontinence. Dorothy Mandelstam, 1977. (Heinemann Medical Books, for the Disabled Living Foundation, London).

Regaining Bladder Control. Eileen Montgomery, 1974. (John Wright & Sons Ltd., Bristol).

Management of Incontinence in the Home: A Survey. Patricia Dobson, 1974. (The Disabled Living Foundation).

Incontinence: A burden for families with handicapped children. Jonathan Bradshaw, 1978. (The Disabled Living Foundation).

Help for Bed Wetting. Roy Meadow, 1980. Churchill Livingstone Patient Handbook (Churchill Livingstone, Edinburgh).

Further advice, including aids and equipment, can be obtained by writing to The Incontinence Advisory Service, The Disabled Living Foundation, 346 Kensington High Street, London W14 8NS. (Enquiries by letter only.)